GUT HEALING REVOLUTION: HARNESSING THE POWER OF PREBIOTICS, PROBIOTICS, AND BUTYRATE FOR OPTIMAL HEALTH AND VITALITY

By

Linda Lewis

Welcome to the wonderful world of prebiotics, probiotics and butyrate. I am about to fascinate you on these 3 remarkable tools to generate a wonderful way to live and create a healthier body.

FIRST, LET US START WITH PREBIOTICS.

History of Prebiotics:

1. **Early Observations (19th Century):**
   - In the 19th century, researchers and scientists began to observe the impact of certain foods on gut health. It was noted that some substances seemed to support digestive well-being, although the mechanisms were not fully understood at that time.

2. **Emergence of the Term "Prebiotics" (1995):**
   - The term "prebiotic" was first introduced in 1995. The definition emphasized the importance of non-digestible food ingredients that positively influence the host by selectively promoting the growth and/or activity of specific bacteria in the colon.

How Prebiotics Work:

1. **Selective Stimulation:**
   - Prebiotics are typically non-digestible fibers or compounds resistant to digestion in the upper gastrointestinal tract. They reach the colon intact, where they selectively stimulate the growth and activity of beneficial bacteria while not supporting the growth of harmful

microbes.

2. **Fermentation Process:**
   - Once in the colon, these prebiotics undergo fermentation by the resident beneficial bacteria. This process results in the production of short-chain fatty acids (SCFAs), such as butyrate, acetate, and propionate. Butyrate, in particular, is known for its positive effects on colonic health.

3. **Health Benefits:**
   - **Digestive Health:** The selective stimulation of beneficial bacteria contributes to a balanced microbiome, aiding in the digestion of complex carbohydrates and promoting overall gut health. Prebiotics can also enhance bowel regularity.

   - **Immune System Support:** A healthy gut microbiome is linked to a robust immune system. Prebiotics indirectly support immune function by contributing to a balanced and diverse microbial community in the gut.

   - **Metabolic Health:** Some studies suggest that prebiotics may have a role in improving metabolic health. They may influence factors such as insulin sensitivity and glucose regulation.

4. **Sources of Prebiotics:**

- **Inulin and Fructooligosaccharides (FOS):** Found in foods like onions, garlic, leeks, and bananas, these fibers are common prebiotics.

- **Galactooligosaccharides (GOS):** Present in foods like legumes and certain grains, GOS also act as prebiotics.

- **Resistant Starch:** Found in unripe bananas, whole grains, and legumes, resistant starch is another type of prebiotic.

5. **Synergy with Probiotics:**

- Prebiotics and probiotics complement each other in promoting gut health. Probiotics are live microorganisms that confer health benefits, while prebiotics provide the necessary nourishment for these beneficial microbes. The combination of prebiotics and probiotics, known as symbiotic, may enhance their respective effects.

Research and Future Directions:

1. **Ongoing Studies:**

- Research on prebiotics is an evolving field, with ongoing studies exploring their specific effects on various aspects of health, including neurological function and mental well-being.

2. **Potential Applications:**
      - Prebiotics are being investigated for their potential applications in personalized nutrition and therapeutic interventions for conditions such as inflammatory bowel disease (IBD) and irritable bowel syndrome (IBS).

In conclusion, the history of prebiotics traces back to early observations of the effects of certain foods on gut health. Today, our understanding has deepened, revealing the selective stimulation of beneficial bacteria in the colon and the resulting health benefits. Prebiotics play a crucial role in maintaining a balanced gut microbiome, supporting digestive health, and influencing broader aspects of well-being.

Ongoing research continues to uncover their full potential and applications in promoting human health.

Second, let us look at probiotics.

History of Probiotics:

1. **Early Observations (20th Century):**
      - The concept of probiotics began to take shape in the early 20th century when scientists observed that certain fermented foods, particularly yogurt, seemed to have positive effects on health. These observations sparked interest in understanding the role of microorganisms in promoting well-being.

2. **Elie Metchnikoff's Contribution (early 20th Century):**
      - Elie Metchnikoff, a Russian immunologist,

is credited with pioneering probiotic research. In the early 1900s, he proposed that the consumption of fermented dairy products containing lactic acid bacteria could contribute to longevity and overall health. His work laid the groundwork for the exploration of the health benefits associated with specific microorganisms.

3. **Isolation and Identification (Late 19th to Mid-20th Century):**

   - Advances in microbiology allowed scientists to isolate and identify microorganisms with probiotic properties. Lactic acid bacteria, including strains of Lactobacillus and Bifidobacterium, became prominent subjects of study. Researchers focused on understanding how these microorganisms interacted with the human body and contributed to health.

4. **Commercialization and Yogurt Industry (20th Century):**

   - The commercialization of probiotics gained traction with the rise of the yogurt industry. Manufacturers began to market products containing live cultures, and the association between probiotics and digestive health became widely recognized. This period saw an increase in the availability and consumption of probiotic-rich foods.

5. **Scientific Advancements (Late 20th Century Onward):**

   - As scientific techniques advanced,

researchers gained a deeper understanding of the mechanisms by which probiotics exert their effects. The development of molecular biology and genomic tools facilitated the identification and characterization of specific strains, allowing for more targeted research on their health benefits.

How Probiotics Work:

1. **Introduction of Beneficial Microorganisms:**
   - Probiotics are live microorganisms, primarily bacteria (such as Lactobacillus and Bifidobacterium species) and yeast (such as Saccharomyces boulardii), which, when consumed in adequate amounts, confer health benefits to the host.

2. **Colonization in the Gut:**
   - After ingestion, probiotics travel through the digestive tract. While some probiotics may temporarily colonize the gut, others exert their effects without establishing a long-term presence. Regular consumption may enhance their potential benefits.

3. **Competitive Exclusion and Microbiota Modulation:**
   - Probiotics contribute to a healthy gut environment by engaging in competitive exclusion. They compete with harmful microorganisms for resources and attachment sites in the gastrointestinal tract. Probiotics may also modulate the overall composition and balance of the gut microbiota.

4. **Production of Bioactive Compounds:**
   - Probiotics produce bioactive compounds, including short-chain fatty acids (SCFAs), antimicrobial peptides, and certain vitamins. SCFAs, such as butyrate, play a crucial role in maintaining gut health and may have systemic effects on the body.

5. **Immunomodulation:**
   - Probiotics interact with the immune system, influencing both innate and adaptive immune responses. They may enhance the body's defense mechanisms against pathogens and contribute to a balanced immune system.

6. **Health Benefits:**
   - **Digestive Health:** Probiotics are well-known for their role in promoting digestive health. They can help maintain a balanced gut microbiome, alleviate symptoms of conditions like irritable bowel syndrome (IBS), and support overall gut function.

   - **Immune Support:** Probiotics may enhance the body's immune response, providing protection against infections and promoting a balanced immune system.

   - **Mental Health:** Emerging research suggests a connection between gut health and mental well-being, with certain probiotics showing potential in influencing mood and cognitive function.

Future Directions and Challenges:

1. **Strain-Specific Effects:**
   - Different probiotic strains may have specific effects on health. Future research aims to identify and understand the properties of individual strains for targeted health interventions.

2. **Personalized Probiotics:**
   - Advances in microbiome research may lead to personalized probiotic recommendations based on an individual's unique microbial profile, optimizing the potential benefits.

In summary, the history of probiotics has evolved from early observations to the identification of specific strains with targeted health benefits. Probiotics work by introducing beneficial microorganisms into the gut, where they influence the microbiota, produce bioactive compounds, and modulate the immune system. Ongoing research continues to unravel the full potential of probiotics and their applications in promoting a healthier body.

Third, let us throw in some information about resistant starches.

History of Naturally Occurring Resistant Starches:

1. **Discovery and Early Observations:**
   - The understanding of resistant starch dates back to the mid-20th century when researchers began to observe that not all dietary starch was fully digested and absorbed in the small intestine. This realization sparked interest in the investigation of starches that resisted enzymatic breakdown during digestion.

2. **Classification and Types of Resistant Starch (1980s Onward):**
   - In the 1980s, scientists started to classify resistant starch into distinct types based on its physical and chemical properties. This classification system includes four main types:
       - **RS1 (Physically Inaccessible Starch):** Found in the outer layers of whole grains, seeds, and legumes, RS1 is physically protected by plant cell walls, making it resistant to digestion.
       - **RS2 (Raw Starch Granules):** Present in raw or uncooked forms of certain foods like potatoes, green bananas, and some legumes, RS2 is resistant due to the crystalline structure of its raw starch granules.
       - **RS3 (Retrograded Starch):** Formed when certain starchy foods, such as potatoes and rice, are cooked and then cooled.
       - The cooling process leads to the retrogradation of starch, making it resistant to digestion.
       - **RS4 (Chemically Modified Starch):** Created through chemical modifications like esterification or cross-linking to enhance resistance. RS4 is often used in food processing.

How Naturally Occurring Resistant Starches Work for a Healthier Body:

1. **Digestive Process:**
   - Resistant starches escape full digestion

in the small intestine, reaching the colon largely intact. This resistance to enzymatic breakdown sets the stage for their unique physiological effects.

2. **Fermentation by Gut Microbiota:**
   - In the colon, resistant starch serves as a substrate for fermentation by beneficial gut bacteria. During this process, microorganisms break down the starch, producing short-chain fatty acids (SCFAs) as byproducts. SCFAs, such as butyrate, acetate, and propionate, are essential for maintaining gut health.

3. **Health Benefits:**
   - **Gut Health:** Resistant starch promotes the growth of beneficial bacteria, such as bifidobacteria and lactobacilli, leading to a balanced and diverse microbiome. This contributes to the overall health of the digestive system and the intestinal lining.

   - **Blood Sugar Regulation:** Resistant starch has been associated with improved insulin sensitivity and better blood sugar control. It can help manage postprandial glucose levels, making it beneficial for individuals with diabetes or those at risk of insulin resistance.

   - **Weight Management:** Some studies suggest that resistant starch may contribute to weight management by increasing feelings of fullness and reducing overall calorie absorption. This can potentially support weight loss efforts.

- **Improved Lipid Profile:** Resistant starch has been linked to favorable changes in lipid metabolism, including lower levels of triglycerides and cholesterol. These effects may contribute to cardiovascular health.

4. **Food Sources:**
    - Natural sources of resistant starch are found in a variety of foods, including whole grains, legumes, green bananas, raw potatoes, and certain cooked and cooled starchy foods like potato salad and sushi rice.

Future Directions and Considerations:

1. **Research Advances:**
    - Ongoing research aims to delve deeper into the specific health effects of different types of resistant starch, considering factors such as dosage, duration of consumption, and individual variations.

2. **Functional Foods and Fortification:**
    - There is a growing interest in incorporating resistant starch into functional foods or fortifying existing products to enhance their health-promoting properties. This could offer consumers convenient ways to increase their intake of resistant starch.

In summary, the history of naturally occurring resistant starches involves the recognition of their resistance to digestion, classification into different types, and the understanding of their potential health benefits. Resistant starch works by resisting digestion in the small intestine, undergoing fermentation in the colon, and contributing to the production of beneficial short-chain fatty acids. Consumption of resistant starch from natural sources is associated with various health benefits, making it an important component of a balanced and healthy diet. Ongoing research continues to uncover the nuances of their effects and potential applications in promoting overall well-being.

Here is a simplified list of foods for the first 3 resistant starches and information on the modified food starch in simplistic terms for your information.

RS1 (Physically Inaccessible Starch):

Found in the outer layers of whole grains, seeds, and legumes, RS1 is physically protected by plant cell walls.

1. **Whole Grains:**
   - Brown rice
   - Quinoa
   - Barley
   - Oats (especially oat bran)
   - Whole wheat

2. **Seeds:**
   - Chia seeds
   - Flaxseeds
   - Sunflower seeds
   - Pumpkin seeds

3. **Legumes:**
   - Lentils

- Chickpeas
- Black beans
- Kidney beans

RS2 (Raw Starch Granules):

Present in raw or uncooked forms of certain foods like potatoes, green bananas, and some legumes, RS2 is resistant due to the crystalline structure of its raw starch granules.

1. **Raw Potatoes:**
   - Raw potato starch

2. **Green Bananas:**
   - Unripe or green bananas

3. **Raw Legumes:**
   - Raw peas
   - Raw lentils

RS3 (Retrograded Starch):

Formed when certain starchy foods, such as potatoes and rice, are cooked and then cooled. The cooling process leads to the retrogradation of starch, making it resistant to digestion.

1. **Cooked and Cooled Potatoes:**
   - Potato salad
   - Cold potato dishes

2. **Cooked and Cooled Rice:**
   - Sushi rice

RS4 (Chemically Modified Starch):

Created through chemical modifications like esterification or cross-linking to enhance resistance. RS4 is often used in food processing.

1. **Chemically Modified Starch (Used in Processed Foods):**
   - Certain processed foods may contain chemically modified starches to improve their texture, stability, or resistance to digestion. Check ingredient labels for specific types of modified starches.

It is important to note that the resistant starch content in these foods can vary based on factors such as preparation methods and cooking techniques. Including a variety of these whole foods in your diet can contribute to a diverse intake of resistant starch and its potential health benefits.

Fourth, let us now look at butyrate.

History of Butyrate:

1. **Discovery and Isolation (19th Century):**
   - In the 19th century, butyrate was first identified and isolated from butter, giving it its name. Early chemists recognized it as a short-chain fatty acid present in various fats and oils.

2. **Physiological Observations (20th Century):**
   - Throughout the 20th century, scientists began to explore the physiological effects of short-chain fatty acids, including butyrate. Early research focused on its presence in the digestive system and its potential impact on health.

3. **Gut Microbiota Connection (Late 20th Century Onward):**
    - The late 20th century marked a shift in understanding as researchers started to investigate the role of gut microbiota in the production of butyrate. It became evident that butyrate is a byproduct of bacterial fermentation, particularly in the colon.

4. **Gut-Brain Axis and Beyond (Recent Decades):**
    - Recent decades have seen increased interest in the gut-brain axis and the broader impact of butyrate beyond the digestive system. Emerging research suggests potential connections between butyrate and neurological functions, mental health, and systemic metabolic benefits.

How Butyrate Works to Make a Healthier Body:

1. **Fermentation by Gut Bacteria:**
    - Butyrate is primarily produced through the fermentation of dietary fibers by specific gut bacteria, including Firmicutes. These bacteria break down complex carbohydrates that reach the colon undigested, producing butyrate as a metabolic byproduct.

2. **Energy Source for Colonocytes:**
    - Colonocytes, the cells lining the colon, utilize butyrate as their primary energy source. This process is crucial for maintaining the health and function of the colon, as it supports the energy needs

of these cells and contributes to the overall integrity of the gut barrier.

3. **Anti-Inflammatory Effects:**
   - Butyrate exhibits anti-inflammatory properties by influencing various cellular processes. It can modulate immune responses in the gut, helping to maintain a balanced and controlled inflammatory environment. This anti-inflammatory action contributes to overall gut health.

4. **Maintenance of Gut Barrier Function:**
   - Butyrate plays a key role in preserving the integrity of the gut barrier. It enhances the production of mucin, a protective layer that lines the gastrointestinal tract, and promotes the tight junctions between epithelial cells. This helps prevent the leakage of harmful substances from the gut into the bloodstream.

5. **Potential Anti-Cancer Effects:**
   - Studies suggest that butyrate may have anti-cancer effects, particularly in the context of colorectal cancer. It influences cellular processes, such as cell differentiation and apoptosis (programmed cell death), and inhibits the growth of cancerous cells.

6. **Metabolic Benefits:**
   - Butyrate has been linked to metabolic benefits, including improved insulin sensitivity. It may play a role in regulating glucose metabolism and supporting overall metabolic health. These effects

have implications for conditions such as insulin resistance and metabolic syndrome.

7. **Neurological Impact:**

- Emerging research indicates a potential connection between butyrate and neurological functions. The gut-brain axis, the bidirectional communication between the gut and the central nervous system, is an area of investigation. Some studies suggest that butyrate may influence brain function and contribute to mental well-being.

Considerations and Future Directions:

1. **Dietary Sources:**

- Dietary fibers found in fruits, vegetables, whole grains, and legumes are crucial for the production of butyrate through bacterial fermentation. Including a diverse range of these foods in the diet promotes a healthy gut microbiome and supports butyrate production.

2. **Supplementation and Therapeutic Potential:**

- Butyrate supplementation is an area of ongoing research, exploring its therapeutic potential in various health conditions, including gastrointestinal disorders and metabolic diseases. However, further studies are needed to determine optimal dosages and specific applications.

In summary, butyrate has a rich history, with its identification in butter laying the foundation for subsequent research. Its role in gut health, energy metabolism, anti-inflammatory actions, and potential systemic benefits make it a critical component for overall well-being. The intricate interplay between dietary factors, gut microbiota, and butyrate production continues to be an active area of scientific exploration.

Ongoing research is expected to uncover additional nuances in the multifaceted roles of butyrate and its impact on human health.

Wow, Wow, Wow! Who knew all this??

This is why I am passing the information along so you can know too. It is also my understanding that if we all eat these foods together in moderation according to each person's own needs etc., (Which I strongly advise you to consult your physician and specialist if you need to figure out the correct path for you because we all unique and not one of us is exactly the same). I am only able to give you a brief overview.

Butyrate is produced through the fermentation of dietary fibers by specific gut bacteria in the colon. Including foods rich in these fibers can promote the production of butyrate. Here is a list of natural foods that are good sources of dietary fibers and can contribute to butyrate production:

Foods Rich in Dietary Fibers:

1. **Whole Grains:**
   - Brown rice
   - Quinoa
   - Oats (especially oat bran)
   - Whole wheat

- Barley

2. **Legumes:**

  - Lentils
  - Chickpeas
  - Black beans
  - Kidney beans

3. **Fruits:**

  - Apples (with skin)
  - Pears (with skin)
  - Berries (strawberries, blueberries, raspberries)
  - Bananas (especially unripe or green bananas)
  - Oranges

4. **Vegetables:**

  - Broccoli
  - Brussels sprouts
  - Carrots
  - Spinach
  - Kale
  - Sweet potatoes

5. **Nuts and Seeds:**

  - Almonds
  - Chia seeds
  - Flaxseeds
  - Sunflower seeds

6. **Whole Vegetables:**

- Garlic
- Onions
- Leeks

7. **Tubers:**
   - Jerusalem artichokes
   - Jicama

8. **Whole Grains and Pseudocereals:**
   - Buckwheat
   - Amaranth

Fermented Foods:

While not directly sources of butyrate, fermented foods may support a healthy gut microbiome, promoting an environment conducive to butyrate production. Some examples include:

1. **Yogurt:** Choose plain, unsweetened yogurt with live and active cultures.

2. **Kefir:** A fermented milk drink containing probiotic bacteria.

3. **Sauerkraut:** Fermented cabbage.

4. **Kimchi:** A traditional Korean dish of fermented vegetables.

Considerations:

- **Diversity:** Aim for a diverse range of fiber-rich foods to promote a varied gut microbiome.

- **Prebiotics:** Some fibers act as prebiotics, promoting the growth of beneficial gut bacteria. In turn, these bacteria may contribute to the production of butyrate.

Incorporating these foods into your diet can support the production of butyrate and contribute to overall gut health. However, individual responses to dietary changes can vary, and it is advisable to introduce these foods gradually to allow your gut microbiome to adjust. If you have specific health concerns or conditions, it is recommended to consult with a healthcare professional or a registered dietitian for personalized advice.

So now you know how good prebiotic, probiotic and butyrate all work together, let us look at some sample daily meal plans. (Be Aware that some of the meals are used again in other meals just mixing it up).

Here is a sample regular meal plan: You can swap other meals within the same category like breakfast to breakfast etc.

DAY 1:

Breakfast:

- Overnight oats with sliced bananas and chia seeds.

Lunch:

- Quinoa salad with mixed vegetables (broccoli, bell peppers, cherry tomatoes) and a lemon-tahini dressing.

Dinner:

- Grilled salmon with steamed asparagus and sweet potato.

DAY 2:

Breakfast:

- Greek yogurt parfait with berries, almonds, and a drizzle of honey.

Lunch:

- Lentil soup with a side of mixed greens and whole-grain bread.

Dinner:

- Stir-fried tofu with bok choy, mushrooms, and brown rice.

DAY 3:

Breakfast:

- Smoothie with kefir, spinach, pineapple, and flaxseeds.

Lunch:

- Chickpea salad with cucumber, tomatoes, feta cheese, and olive oil.

Dinner:

- Grilled chicken breast with roasted Brussels sprouts and quinoa.

DAY 4:

Breakfast:

- Whole grain toast with avocado and poached eggs.

Lunch:

- Spinach and feta stuffed bell peppers with a side of hummus and carrot sticks.

Dinner:

- Baked cod with lemon and herbs, served with a side of sautéed kale and wild rice.

DAY 5:

Breakfast:

- Oatmeal topped with sliced apples, walnuts, and a sprinkle of cinnamon.

Lunch:

- Brown rice bowl with black beans, corn, salsa, and guacamole.

Dinner:

- Beef and vegetable kebabs with quinoa pilaf.

DAY 6:

Breakfast:

- Cottage cheese with sliced peaches and a handful of almonds.

Lunch:

- Tomato and basil whole grain pasta with a side of mixed greens.

Dinner:

- Grilled shrimp with roasted sweet potatoes and green beans.

DAY 7:

Breakfast:

- Whole grain pancakes with blueberries and a dollop of yogurt.

Lunch:

- Quinoa and black bean stuffed bell peppers with a side of Greek salad.

Dinner:

- Turkey chili with kidney beans, tomatoes, and a sprinkle of cheese.

Repeat this cycle for the following days, incorporating a variety of fruits, vegetables, whole grains, lean proteins, and fermented foods. Adjust portion sizes based on individual nutritional needs. Remember to stay hydrated and consider consulting with a healthcare professional or a registered dietitian for personalized advice based on specific dietary requirements or health conditions.

DAY 8:

Breakfast:

- Smoothie with kefir, banana, spinach, and a scoop of ground flaxseeds.

Lunch:

- Quinoa and black bean salad with diced tomatoes, corn, and a lime vinaigrette.

Dinner:

- Grilled chicken breast with a side of roasted sweet potatoes and steamed broccoli.

DAY 9:

Breakfast:

- Whole grain toast with mashed avocado, poached eggs, and a sprinkle of chia seeds.

Lunch:

- Lentil and vegetable curry served over brown rice.

Dinner:

- Baked salmon with a dill and lemon sauce, accompanied by quinoa and sautéed spinach.

DAY 10:

Breakfast:

- Overnight chia seed pudding made with almond milk, topped with mixed berries.

Lunch:

- Chickpea and vegetable stir-fry with tofu, broccoli, and snap peas over brown rice.

Dinner:

- Turkey and vegetable skewers with a side of wild rice and a green salad.

DAY 11:

Breakfast:

- Cottage cheese and pineapple parfait with a handful of walnuts.

Lunch:

- Whole grain wrap with hummus, falafel, cucumber, tomatoes, and a drizzle of tahini.

Dinner:

- Beef and vegetable stir-fry with a variety of colorful vegetables served over quinoa.

DAY 12:

Breakfast:

- Oatmeal with sliced strawberries, almonds, and a drizzle of honey.

Lunch:

- Whole grain pasta salad with cherry tomatoes, olives, feta cheese, and an olive oil dressing.

Dinner:

- Grilled shrimp with garlic and herbs, paired with sweet potato wedges and sautéed kale.

DAY 13:

Breakfast:

- Greek yogurt bowl with mango, granola, and a sprinkle of sunflower seeds.

Lunch:

- Black bean and vegetable burrito bowl with brown rice, salsa, guacamole, and a dollop of yogurt.

Dinner:

- Baked cod with a tomato and olive salsa, served with quinoa and roasted Brussels sprouts.

DAY 14:

Breakfast:

- Whole grain pancakes with sliced peaches and a dollop of Greek yogurt.

Lunch:

- Quinoa and lentil stuffed bell peppers with a side of mixed greens.

Dinner:

- Turkey and vegetable chili with a side of whole grain cornbread.

Repeat this cycle for the next set of days, maintaining a balance of prebiotic-rich foods (fiber), probiotics (fermented foods), and considering foods that support butyrate production. Adjust the plan based on individual preferences and dietary needs.

Always stay hydrated, and for personalized advice, consider consulting with a healthcare professional or a registered dietitian.

DAY 15:

Breakfast:

- Smoothie with kefir, mixed berries, spinach, and a tablespoon of ground flaxseeds.

Lunch:

- Chickpea and spinach curry with whole grain naan bread.

Dinner:

- Grilled chicken thighs with a lemon-rosemary marinade, accompanied by roasted sweet potatoes and green beans.

DAY 16:

Breakfast:

- Whole grain toast with smoked salmon, cream cheese, and sliced cucumbers.

Lunch:

- Lentil and vegetable soup with a side of quinoa and a mixed green salad.

Dinner:

- Baked tilapia with a mango salsa, served with wild rice and steamed broccoli.

DAY 17:

Breakfast:

- Greek yogurt parfait with granola, kiwi slices, and a drizzle of honey.

Lunch:

- Whole grain wrap with hummus, roasted vegetables, feta cheese, and a handful of olives.

Dinner:

- Stir-fried tofu with a ginger-soy glaze, paired with brown rice and sautéed bok choy.

DAY 18:

Breakfast:

- Overnight chia seed pudding made with almond milk, topped with sliced bananas and chopped walnuts.

Lunch:

- Quinoa salad with black beans, corn, avocado, and a lime-cilantro dressing.

Dinner:

- Grilled shrimp skewers with a pineapple and bell pepper salsa, served with quinoa.

DAY 19:

Breakfast:

- Oatmeal with diced apples, cinnamon, and a dollop of Greek yogurt.

Lunch:

- Black bean and vegetable burritos with whole grain tortillas, salsa, guacamole, and a side of mixed greens.

Dinner:

- Baked chicken breast with a rosemary and garlic marinade, accompanied by sweet potato wedges and roasted Brussels sprouts.

DAY 20:

Breakfast:

- Cottage cheese and berry bowl with a sprinkle of sunflower seeds.

Lunch:

- Whole grain pasta with cherry tomatoes, spinach, garlic, and olive oil, topped with grated Parmesan cheese.

Dinner:

- Turkey and vegetable stir-fry with a variety of colorful vegetables over quinoa.

DAY 21:

Breakfast:

- Whole grain pancakes with blueberries, sliced almonds, and a dollop of yogurt.

Lunch:

- Lentil and vegetable wrap with hummus, cucumber, and a squeeze of lemon.

Dinner:

- Grilled salmon with a dill and lemon sauce, served with brown rice and steamed broccoli.

Adjust portion sizes based on individual needs and preferences. Staying hydrated and incorporating physical activity into your routine can further contribute to overall well-being. If you have specific dietary concerns or health conditions, consider consulting with a healthcare professional or a registered dietitian for personalized guidance.

DAY 22:

Breakfast:

- Smoothie with kefir, mango, spinach, and a tablespoon of chia seeds.

Lunch:

- Quinoa and black bean bowl with avocado, salsa, and a dollop of Greek yogurt.

Dinner:

- Grilled chicken thighs with a Mediterranean-inspired quinoa salad (tomatoes, cucumbers, olives, feta).

DAY 23:

Breakfast:

- Whole grain toast with mashed avocado, poached eggs, and a sprinkle of pumpkin seeds.

Lunch:

- Lentil and vegetable stir-fry with tofu, broccoli, and brown rice.

Dinner:

- Baked cod with a lemon and herb crust, served with sweet potato wedges and steamed asparagus.

DAY 24:

Breakfast:

- Greek yogurt parfait with granola, mixed berries, and a drizzle of honey.

Lunch:

- Chickpea and spinach stuffed bell peppers with a side of quinoa.

Dinner:

- Stir-fried tofu with a teriyaki glaze, paired with brown rice and sautéed bok choy.

DAY 25:

Breakfast:

- Oatmeal with sliced strawberries, almonds, and a dollop of Greek yogurt.

Lunch:

- Black bean and vegetable burrito bowl with brown rice, salsa, guacamole, and a dollop of yogurt.

Dinner:

- Grilled shrimp with garlic and lemon, served with quinoa and roasted Brussels sprouts.

DAY 26:

Breakfast:

- Cottage cheese and pineapple bowl with a sprinkle of chia seeds.

Lunch:

- Whole grain wrap with hummus, roasted vegetables, feta cheese, and olives.

Dinner:

- Turkey and vegetable chili with a side of whole grain cornbread.

DAY 27:

Breakfast:

- Smoothie with kefir, mixed berries, spinach, and a tablespoon of ground flaxseeds.

Lunch:

- Quinoa and lentil stuffed bell peppers with a side of mixed greens.

Dinner:

- Baked salmon with a dill and lemon sauce, accompanied by quinoa and sautéed spinach.

DAY 28:

Breakfast:

- Whole grain pancakes with sliced peaches and a dollop of Greek yogurt.

Lunch:

- Tomato and basil whole grain pasta with a side of mixed greens.

Dinner:

- Grilled shrimp with garlic and herbs, paired with sweet potato wedges and sautéed kale.

Adjust the plan based on individual preferences and dietary needs. Always stay hydrated, and for personalized advice, consider consulting with a healthcare professional or a registered dietitian.

DAY 29:

Breakfast:

- Whole grain toast with smoked salmon, cream cheese, and sliced cucumbers.

Lunch:

- Lentil and vegetable soup with a side of quinoa and a mixed green salad.

Dinner:

- Baked tilapia with a mango salsa, served with wild rice and steamed broccoli.

DAY 30:

Breakfast:

- Greek yogurt bowl with mango, granola, and a sprinkle of sunflower seeds.

Lunch:

- Black bean and vegetable burritos with whole grain tortillas, salsa, guacamole, and a side of mixed greens.

Dinner:

- Stir-fried tofu with a ginger-soy glaze, paired with brown rice and sautéed bok choy.

DAY 31: (VARIATION)

Breakfast:

- Overnight chia seed pudding made with almond milk, topped with sliced bananas and chopped walnuts.

Lunch:

- Quinoa salad with black beans, corn, avocado, and a lime-cilantro dressing.

Dinner:

- Grilled shrimp skewers with a pineapple and bell pepper salsa, served with quinoa.

Notes:

- **Fluid Intake:** Ensure adequate water intake throughout the day to stay hydrated, support digestion, and facilitate nutrient absorption.

- **Snacks:** Incorporate healthy snacks like raw vegetables with hummus, a piece of fruit, or a small handful of nuts between meals.

- **Probiotic Sources:** Consider adding fermented foods like yogurt, kefir, sauerkraut, or kimchi as snacks or in meals for additional probiotic benefits.

- **Exercise:** Combine this meal plan with regular physical activity for overall health and well-being.

Remember that individual dietary needs and preferences vary, so feel free to adjust the plan based on your specific requirements. If you have any health concerns or conditions, it is advisable to consult with a healthcare professional or a registered dietitian for personalized guidance.

Here is a sample daily menu for vegans. Fill free to mix and match like above, We Don't judge.

DAY 1: BREAKFAST:

- Chia Seed Pudding made with almond milk, topped with berries and sliced almonds.

- Probiotic: Vegan coconut yogurt.

Lunch:

- Quinoa Salad with mixed vegetables (bell peppers, cucumber, cherry tomatoes).

- Prebiotic: Chicory greens or arugula.

- Probiotic: Sauerkraut.

Dinner:

- Baked Tofu with Steamed Broccoli and Asparagus.

- Prebiotic: Garlic-roasted Brussels sprouts.

- Probiotic: Kimchi.

Snack:

- Raw Carrot Sticks with Hummus.

DAY 2: BREAKFAST:

- Smoothie with spinach, avocado, almond milk, and a handful of blueberries.

- Probiotic: Vegan probiotic supplement.

Lunch:

- Zucchini Noodles with Pesto (made with basil, pine nuts, nutritional yeast, and olive oil).

- Prebiotic: Raw jicama sticks.

- Probiotic: Coconut kefir.

Dinner:

- Lentil and Vegetable Stew.

- Prebiotic: Onions and leeks.

- Probiotic: Vegan miso soup.

Snack:

- Handful of Almonds.

Remember to drink plenty of water throughout the day and adjust portion sizes as needed. It's crucial to listen to your body and make modifications based on your energy levels, hunger, and overall well-being. Additionally, consider consulting with a healthcare professional or a registered dietitian to ensure that this meal plan meets your specific nutritional needs.

DAY 3: BREAKFAST:

- Oatmeal made with water, topped with sliced bananas and a sprinkle of flaxseeds.
- Probiotic: Vegan coconut or almond yogurt.

Lunch:

- Stir-Fried Tofu with Bell Peppers and Snap Peas.
- Prebiotic: Sautéed onions and garlic.
- Probiotic: Pickles or pickled cucumbers.

Dinner:

- Chickpea and Spinach Curry.
- Prebiotic: Cooked and chilled potatoes (resistant starch).
- Probiotic: Vegan yogurt raita.

Snack:

- Celery Sticks with Peanut Butter.

DAY 4: BREAKFAST:

- Whole Grain Toast with Avocado and Cherry Tomatoes.

- Probiotic: Vegan kimchi.

Lunch:

- Cauliflower Rice Bowl with Black Beans, Corn, and Salsa.

- Prebiotic: Shredded cabbage.

- Probiotic: Vegan sour cream.

Dinner:

- Baked Eggplant with Tomato Sauce and Vegan Cheese.

- Prebiotic: Cooked and cooled quinoa.

- Probiotic: Pickled jalapeños.

Snack:

- Apple Slices with Almond Butter.

DAY 5: BREAKFAST:

- Vegan Protein Smoothie with Spinach, Berries, and Plant-Based Protein Powder.

- Probiotic: Vegan probiotic supplement.

Lunch:

- Spinach and Mushroom Salad with Lemon-Tahini Dressing.

- Prebiotic: Raw radishes.

- Probiotic: Fermented olives.

Dinner:

- Portobello Mushroom "Steak" with Roasted Asparagus.

- Prebiotic: Sautéed onions.

- Probiotic: Vegan sauerkraut.

Snack:

- Handful of Walnuts.

These meal ideas are designed to be cost-effective and use ingredients that are commonly available. Adjust portion sizes based on your individual needs and consider incorporating a variety of foods to ensure a well-rounded nutrient intake. Remember, consulting with a healthcare professional or a registered dietitian is advisable to tailor the plan to your specific requirements and to monitor your health throughout the process.

DAY 6: BREAKFAST:

- Vegan Tofu Scramble with Spinach and Cherry Tomatoes.
- Probiotic: Vegan probiotic supplement.

Lunch:

- Cabbage and Carrot Slaw with Lemon-Tahini Dressing.
- Prebiotic: Shredded carrots.
- Probiotic: Vegan coconut yogurt.

Dinner:

- Broccoli and Cauliflower Stir-Fry with Tempeh.
- Prebiotic: Green onions.
- Probiotic: Fermented pickles.

Snack:

- Cucumber Slices with Guacamole.

DAY 7: BREAKFAST:

- Overnight Chia Seed Pudding with Almond Milk, topped with Kiwi and Pomegranate Seeds.

- Probiotic: Vegan coconut or almond yogurt.

Lunch:

- Lentil Salad with Mixed Greens and Balsamic Vinaigrette.

- Prebiotic: Raw bell peppers.

- Probiotic: Vegan sauerkraut.

Dinner:

- Spaghetti Squash with Tomato and Basil Sauce.

- Prebiotic: Sautéed garlic.

- Probiotic: Vegan probiotic supplement.

Snack:

- Roasted Pumpkin Seeds.

Remember to rotate your food choices to ensure a diverse nutrient intake. This meal plan provides a mix of fiber-rich prebiotics, probiotics for gut health, and low-carb vegan options. You can customize the plan based on your taste preferences and any specific nutritional requirements you may have. Additionally, staying hydrated and incorporating a variety of herbs and spices into your meals can add flavor without extra calories. Always keep in mind that individual nutritional needs vary, and it's essential to monitor your health and make any adjustments as needed. If you have any underlying health conditions or specific dietary concerns, it's advisable to consult with a healthcare professional or a registered dietitian for personalized advice.

DAY 8: BREAKFAST:

- Berry and Kale Smoothie with Plant-Based Protein Powder.

- Probiotic: Vegan coconut or almond yogurt.

Lunch:

- Avocado and Black Bean Salad with Lime Vinaigrette.

- Prebiotic: Sliced radishes.

- Probiotic: Fermented pickles.

Dinner:

- Stuffed Bell Peppers with Quinoa, Black Beans, and Salsa.

- Prebiotic: Chopped green onions.

- Probiotic: Vegan sour cream.

Snack:

- Cherry Tomatoes with Hummus.

DAY 9: BREAKFAST:

- Almond Flour Pancakes with Berries and Maple Syrup.
- Probiotic: Vegan probiotic supplement.

Lunch:

- Grilled Portobello Mushroom Wraps with Lettuce and Tomatoes.
- Prebiotic: Sliced cucumber.
- Probiotic: Vegan kimchi.

Dinner:

- Cauliflower and Chickpea Coconut Curry.
- Prebiotic: Sautéed onions and garlic.
- Probiotic: Coconut yogurt.

Snack:

- Sliced Peaches with a Sprinkle of Chia Seeds.

DAY 10: BREAKFAST:

- Vegan Overnight Oats with Almond Milk, topped with Sliced Banana and Almond Butter.

- Probiotic: Vegan coconut or almond yogurt.

Lunch:

- Spinach and Artichoke Stuffed Portobello Mushrooms.

- Prebiotic: Chopped green onions.

- Probiotic: Fermented olives.

Dinner:

- Zucchini and Eggplant Lasagna with Vegan Cheese.

- Prebiotic: Sautéed garlic.

- Probiotic: Vegan sauerkraut.

Snack:

- Raw Bell Pepper Strips with Guacamole.

Feel free to mix and match these meal ideas, and adjust portions as needed to meet your energy requirements. Remember to stay hydrated and, if necessary, consider supplementing with vitamins and minerals to ensure you meet your nutritional needs, especially when following a restrictive diet. Always consult with a healthcare professional or a registered dietitian for personalized advice based on your specific health conditions and goals.

DAY 11: BREAKFAST:

- Coconut Flour Pancakes with Fresh Strawberries and a Drizzle of Agave Nectar.

- Probiotic: Vegan probiotic supplement.

Lunch:

- Cucumber and Avocado Nori Rolls with Sesame Ginger Dipping Sauce.

- Prebiotic: Shredded carrots.

- Probiotic: Vegan miso soup.

Dinner:

- Stuffed Acorn Squash with Quinoa, Black Beans, and Salsa.

- Prebiotic: Sautéed onions and garlic.

- Probiotic: Vegan coconut yogurt.

Snack:

- Mixed Berries with a Handful of Almonds.

DAY 12: BREAKFAST:

- Green Smoothie Bowl with Kale, Pineapple, and Plant-Based Protein Powder.

- Probiotic: Vegan coconut or almond yogurt.

Lunch:

- Spaghetti Squash Primavera with Tomato and Basil Sauce.

- Prebiotic: Sliced bell peppers.

- Probiotic: Fermented pickles.

Dinner:

- Lentil and Vegetable Stir-Fry with Cauliflower Rice.

- Prebiotic: Chopped green onions.

- Probiotic: Vegan sauerkraut.

Snack:

- Celery Sticks with Peanut Butter.

DAY 13: BREAKFAST:

- Blueberry Almond Flour Muffins.
- Probiotic: Vegan probiotic supplement.

Lunch:

- Chickpea Salad Lettuce Wraps with Tahini Dressing.
- Prebiotic: Sliced radishes.
- Probiotic: Vegan coconut yogurt.

Dinner:

- Baked Sweet Potato with Black Bean and Corn Salsa.
- Prebiotic: Sautéed garlic.
- Probiotic: Vegan kimchi.

Snack:

- Cherry Tomatoes with Hummus.

Feel free to adapt these meal ideas based on your taste preferences and nutritional needs. Additionally, consider incorporating a variety of herbs and spices to enhance the flavor of your meals. It's crucial to monitor your health and make any adjustments as needed. If you have any underlying health conditions or specific dietary concerns, consult with a healthcare professional or a registered dietitian for personalized advice.

DAY 14: BREAKFAST:

- Quinoa Breakfast Bowl with Mixed Berries and Almond Butter.
- Probiotic: Vegan coconut or almond yogurt.

Lunch:

- Broccoli and Almond Salad with Lemon-Tahini Dressing.
- Prebiotic: Raw radishes.
- Probiotic: Vegan miso soup.

Dinner:

- Portobello Mushroom Fajitas with Guacamole.
- Prebiotic: Sliced onions and bell peppers.
- Probiotic: Fermented pickles.

Snack:

- Raw Carrot Sticks with Hummus.

DAY 15: BREAKFAST:

- Smoothie with Spinach, Frozen Berries, and Plant-Based Protein Powder.

- Probiotic: Vegan probiotic supplement.

Lunch:

- Cauliflower and Chickpea Salad with Lemon Vinaigrette.

- Prebiotic: Cherry tomatoes.

- Probiotic: Vegan coconut yogurt.

Dinner:

- Zucchini Noodles with Pesto (nutritional yeast, pine nuts, basil).

- Prebiotic: Sautéed garlic.

- Probiotic: Vegan sauerkraut.

Snack:

- Mixed Berries with a Handful of Walnuts.

DAY 16: BREAKFAST:

- Vegan Protein Pancakes with Sliced Banana and Almond Butter.
- Probiotic: Vegan coconut or almond yogurt.

Lunch:

- Cabbage and Lentil Soup.
- Prebiotic: Chopped green onions.
- Probiotic: Vegan kimchi.

Dinner:

- Stuffed Bell Peppers with Cauliflower Rice, Black Beans, and Salsa.
- Prebiotic: Sautéed onions and garlic.
- Probiotic: Vegan coconut yogurt.

Snack:

- Cucumber Slices with Guacamole.

Remember to drink plenty of water throughout the day, and adjust portion sizes based on your individual needs. Continue to rotate food choices to ensure a diverse nutrient intake. If you have any specific dietary requirements or health concerns, it's advisable to consult with a healthcare professional or a registered dietitian for personalized guidance.

DAY 17: BREAKFAST:

- Berry and Spinach Smoothie Bowl with Chia Seeds.
- Probiotic: Vegan probiotic supplement.

Lunch:

- Stuffed Avocado with Chickpea Salad (cherry tomatoes, cucumber, red onion).
- Prebiotic: Sliced radishes.
- Probiotic: Vegan miso soup.

Dinner:

- Spaghetti Squash with Tomato and Basil Sauce, topped with Nutritional Yeast.
- Prebiotic: Sautéed garlic.
- Probiotic: Vegan sauerkraut.

Snack:

- Apple Slices with Almond Butter.

DAY 18: BREAKFAST:

- Vegan Overnight Oats with Almond Milk, topped with Sliced Peaches and Chopped Almonds.

- Probiotic: Vegan coconut or almond yogurt.

Lunch:

- Cauliflower and Kale Salad with Tahini Dressing.

- Prebiotic: Cherry tomatoes.

- Probiotic: Fermented pickles.

Dinner:

- Lentil and Vegetable Stir-Fry with Quinoa.

- Prebiotic: Chopped green onions.

- Probiotic: Vegan coconut yogurt.

Snack:

- Raw Bell Pepper Strips with Hummus.

DAY 19: BREAKFAST:

- Almond Flour Waffles with Mixed Berries and a Drizzle of Maple Syrup.
- Probiotic: Vegan probiotic supplement.

Lunch:

- Zucchini Noodles with Pesto (nutritional yeast, pine nuts, basil).
- Prebiotic: Sautéed garlic.
- Probiotic: Vegan kimchi.

Dinner:

- Baked Eggplant with Tomato Sauce and Vegan Cheese.
- Prebiotic: Sliced onions.
- Probiotic: Fermented pickles.

Snack:

- Mixed Berries with a Handful of Walnuts.

DAY 20: BREAKFAST:

- Smoothie with Kale, Pineapple, and Plant-Based Protein Powder.
- Probiotic: Vegan coconut or almond yogurt.

Lunch:

- Stuffed Bell Peppers with Quinoa, Black Beans, and Salsa.
- Prebiotic: Chopped green onions.
- Probiotic: Vegan sauerkraut.

Dinner:

- Cauliflower Rice Bowl with Tofu and Mixed Vegetables.
- Prebiotic: Sautéed garlic.
- Probiotic: Vegan coconut yogurt.

Snack:

- Celery Sticks with Peanut Butter.

Remember to customize the plan based on your preferences, and listen to your body's signals regarding hunger and fullness. If you have specific dietary needs or health concerns, it's essential to consult with a healthcare professional or a registered dietitian for personalized advice.

DAY 21: BREAKFAST:

- Chia Seed Pudding made with Almond Milk, topped with Sliced Kiwi and Pomegranate Seeds.
- Probiotic: Vegan coconut or almond yogurt.

Lunch:

- Spinach and Mushroom Stuffed Bell Peppers.
- Prebiotic: Sautéed onions and garlic.
- Probiotic: Vegan kimchi.

Dinner:

- Baked Portobello Mushrooms with Quinoa and Roasted Brussels Sprouts.
- Prebiotic: Sliced onions.
- Probiotic: Vegan sauerkraut.

Snack:

- Raw Carrot Sticks with Hummus.

DAY 22: BREAKFAST:

- Vegan Protein Smoothie with Spinach, Berries, and Plant-Based Protein Powder.
- Probiotic: Vegan probiotic supplement.

Lunch:

- Cucumber Noodles with Avocado Pesto.
- Prebiotic: Sliced radishes.
- Probiotic: Fermented pickles.

Dinner:

- Lentil and Vegetable Curry with Cauliflower Rice.
- Prebiotic: Chopped green onions.
- Probiotic: Vegan coconut yogurt.

Snack:

- Apple Slices with Almond Butter.

DAY 23: BREAKFAST:

- Vegan Omelete with Spinach, Tomatoes, and Vegan Cheese.
- Probiotic: Vegan coconut or almond yogurt.

Lunch:

- Grilled Eggplant and Zucchini Salad with Lemon-Tahini Dressing.
- Prebiotic: Cherry tomatoes.
- Probiotic: Vegan miso soup.

Dinner:

- Stuffed Acorn Squash with Quinoa, Black Beans, and Salsa.
- Prebiotic: Sautéed garlic.
- Probiotic: Vegan sauerkraut.

Snack:

- Mixed Berries with a Handful of Walnuts.

DAY 24: BREAKFAST:

- Blueberry Almond Flour Muffins.

- Probiotic: Vegan probiotic supplement.

Lunch:

- Chickpea Salad Lettuce Wraps with Tahini Dressing.

- Prebiotic: Shredded carrots.

- Probiotic: Vegan coconut yogurt.

Dinner:

- Spaghetti Squash Primavera with Tomato and Basil Sauce.

- Prebiotic: Sautéed garlic.

- Probiotic: Vegan sauerkraut.

Snack:

- Celery Sticks with Peanut Butter.

DAY 25: BREAKFAST:

- Green Smoothie Bowl with Kale, Pineapple, and Plant-Based Protein Powder.

- Probiotic: Vegan coconut or almond yogurt.

Lunch:

- Cauliflower and Chickpea Salad with Lemon Vinaigrette.

- Prebiotic: Sliced cucumber.

- Probiotic: Fermented pickles.

Dinner:

- Zucchini Noodles with Pesto (nutritional yeast, pine nuts, basil).

- Prebiotic: Sautéed garlic.

- Probiotic: Vegan kimchi.

Snack:

- Raw Bell Pepper Strips with Hummus.

DAY 26: BREAKFAST:

- Almond Flour Waffles with Mixed Berries and a Drizzle of Maple Syrup.
- Probiotic: Vegan probiotic supplement.

Lunch:

- Cabbage and Lentil Soup.
- Prebiotic: Chopped green onions.
- Probiotic: Vegan sauerkraut.

Dinner:

- Stuffed Bell Peppers with Cauliflower Rice, Black Beans, and Salsa.
- Prebiotic: Sautéed onions and garlic.
- Probiotic: Vegan coconut yogurt.

Snack:

- Cucumber Slices with Guacamole.

DAY 27: BREAKFAST:

- Vegan Overnight Oats with Almond Milk, topped with Sliced Peaches and Chopped Almonds.
- Probiotic: Vegan coconut or almond yogurt.

Lunch:

- Zucchini Noodles with Avocado Pesto.
- Prebiotic: Sautéed garlic.
- Probiotic: Vegan kimchi.

Dinner:

- Baked Eggplant with Tomato Sauce and Vegan Cheese.
- Prebiotic: Sliced onions.
- Probiotic: Fermented pickles.

Snack:

- Mixed Berries with a Handful of Walnuts.

DAY 28: BREAKFAST:

- Smoothie with Spinach, Frozen Berries, and Plant-Based Protein Powder.
- Probiotic: Vegan probiotic supplement.

Lunch:

- Stuffed Bell Peppers with Quinoa, Black Beans, and Salsa.
- Prebiotic: Chopped green onions.
- Probiotic: Vegan sauerkraut.

Dinner:

- Cauliflower Rice Bowl with Tofu and Mixed Vegetables.
- Prebiotic: Sautéed garlic.
- Probiotic: Vegan coconut yogurt.

Snack:

- Celery Sticks with Peanut Butter.

DAY 29: BREAKFAST:

- Chia Seed Pudding made with Almond Milk, topped with Sliced Kiwi and Pomegranate Seeds.

- Probiotic: Vegan coconut or almond yogurt.

Lunch:

- Spinach and Mushroom Stuffed Bell Peppers.

- Prebiotic: Sautéed onions and garlic.

- Probiotic: Vegan kimchi.

Dinner:

- Baked Portobello Mushrooms with Quinoa and Roasted Brussels Sprouts.

- Prebiotic: Sliced onions.

- Probiotic: Vegan sauerkraut.

Snack:

- Raw Carrot Sticks with Hummus.

DAY 30: BREAKFAST:

- Quinoa Breakfast Bowl with Mixed Berries and Almond Butter.

- Probiotic: Vegan coconut or almond yogurt.

Lunch:

- Broccoli and Almond Salad with Lemon-Tahini Dressing.

- Prebiotic: Raw radishes.

- Probiotic: Vegan miso soup.

Dinner:

- Portobello Mushroom Fajitas with Guacamole.

- Prebiotic: Sliced onions and bell peppers.

- Probiotic: Fermented pickles.

Snack:

- Raw Carrot Sticks with Hummus.

Feel free to adjust portion sizes based on your individual needs and preferences. Additionally, consider incorporating a variety of herbs and spices into your meals to add flavor without extra calories. Remember to stay hydrated throughout the day. If you have specific dietary requirements or health concerns, it's crucial to consult with a healthcare professional or a registered dietitian for personalized advice.

DAY 31: BREAKFAST:

- Vegan Protein Smoothie with Kale, Pineapple, and Plant-Based Protein Powder.

- Probiotic: Vegan coconut or almond yogurt.

Lunch:

- Avocado and Black Bean Salad with Lime Vinaigrette.

- Prebiotic: Sliced radishes.

- Probiotic: Vegan miso soup.

Dinner:

- Stuffed Bell Peppers with Quinoa, Black Beans, and Salsa.

- Prebiotic: Chopped green onions.

- Probiotic: Vegan sauerkraut.

Snack:

- Mixed Berries with a Handful of Almonds.

Remember, this meal plan is just a guide, and you can mix and match these meal ideas based on your preferences. It's important to listen to your body and make any adjustments as needed. Also, ensure that you're meeting your nutritional needs by including a variety of nutrient-dense foods.

Additionally, consider incorporating other sources of butyrate, such as certain types of nuts, seeds, and oils. While the meal plan includes a variety of prebiotic and probiotic foods, it's essential to focus on overall dietary variety for optimal health.

If you have specific health concerns, dietary restrictions, or if you're considering a major dietary change, it's highly recommended to consult with a healthcare professional or a registered dietitian.

They can provide personalized advice based on your individual needs and ensure that you're meeting all your nutritional requirements.

DAY 32: BREAKFAST:

- Chia Seed Pudding made with Almond Milk, topped with Sliced Strawberries and a sprinkle of Flaxseeds.

- Probiotic: Vegan coconut or almond yogurt.

Lunch:

- Grilled Portobello Mushrooms with a Quinoa and Vegetable Stuffing.

- Prebiotic: Sautéed garlic.

- Probiotic: Vegan kimchi.

Dinner:

- Cauliflower Fried Rice with Tofu and Mixed Vegetables.

- Prebiotic: Chopped green onions.

- Probiotic: Vegan coconut yogurt.

Snack:

- Raw Carrot Sticks with Hummus.

DAY 33: BREAKFAST:

- Vegan Protein Pancakes with Sliced Banana and Almond Butter.

- Probiotic: Vegan probiotic supplement.

Lunch:

- Zucchini Noodles with Pesto (nutritional yeast, pine nuts, basil).

- Prebiotic: Sautéed garlic.

- Probiotic: Fermented pickles.

Dinner:

- Stuffed Acorn Squash with Quinoa, Chickpeas, and Roasted Brussels Sprouts.

- Prebiotic: Sliced onions.

- Probiotic: Vegan sauerkraut.

Snack:

- Apple Slices with Almond Butter.

DAY 34: BREAKFAST:

- Smoothie with Spinach, Mixed Berries, and Plant-Based Protein Powder.
- Probiotic: Vegan coconut or almond yogurt.

Lunch:

- Chickpea Salad Lettuce Wraps with Tahini Dressing.
- Prebiotic: Shredded carrots.
- Probiotic: Vegan miso soup.

Dinner:

- Lentil and Vegetable Stir-Fry with Cauliflower Rice.
- Prebiotic: Chopped green onions.
- Probiotic: Vegan coconut yogurt.

Snack:

- Cucumber Slices with Guacamole.

DAY 35: BREAKFAST:

- Vegan Omelete with Spinach, Tomatoes, and Vegan Cheese.
- Probiotic: Vegan coconut or almond yogurt.

Lunch:

- Cabbage and Lentil Soup.
- Prebiotic: Chopped green onions.
- Probiotic: Vegan kimchi.

Dinner:

- Stuffed Bell Peppers with Cauliflower Rice, Black Beans, and Salsa.
- Prebiotic: Sautéed onions and garlic.
- Probiotic: Vegan coconut yogurt.

Snack:

- Raw Bell Pepper Strips with Hummus.

DAY 36: BREAKFAST:

- Almond Flour Waffles with Mixed Berries and a Drizzle of Maple Syrup.

- Probiotic: Vegan probiotic supplement.

Lunch:

- Broccoli and Almond Salad with Lemon-Tahini Dressing.

- Prebiotic: Raw radishes.

- Probiotic: Fermented pickles.

Dinner:

- Baked Eggplant with Tomato Sauce and Vegan Cheese.

- Prebiotic: Sliced onions.

- Probiotic: Vegan sauerkraut.

Snack:

- Mixed Berries with a Handful of Walnuts.

Feel free to customize this meal plan based on your preferences and nutritional needs. Also, consider incorporating a variety of herbs and spices to add flavor to your meals without extra calories. If you have specific dietary requirements or health concerns, it's essential to consult with a healthcare professional or a registered dietitian for personalized advice.

DAY 37: BREAKFAST:

- Quinoa Breakfast Bowl with Mixed Berries and Almond Butter.

- Probiotic: Vegan coconut or almond yogurt.

Lunch:

- Stuffed Bell Peppers with Quinoa, Black Beans, and Salsa.

- Prebiotic: Chopped green onions.

- Probiotic: Vegan sauerkraut.

Dinner:

- Cauliflower Rice Bowl with Tofu and Mixed Vegetables.

- Prebiotic: Sautéed garlic.

- Probiotic: Vegan coconut yogurt.

Snack:

- Celery Sticks with Peanut Butter.

DAY 38: BREAKFAST:

- Chia Seed Pudding made with Almond Milk, topped with Sliced Kiwi and Pomegranate Seeds.
- Probiotic: Vegan coconut or almond yogurt.

Lunch:

- Grilled Portobello Mushrooms with a Quinoa and Vegetable Stuffing.
- Prebiotic: Sautéed garlic.
- Probiotic: Vegan kimchi.

Dinner:

- Lentil and Vegetable Curry with Cauliflower Rice.
- Prebiotic: Chopped green onions.
- Probiotic: Vegan coconut yogurt.

Snack:

- Raw Carrot Sticks with Hummus.

DAY 39: BREAKFAST:

- Vegan Protein Smoothie with Kale, Pineapple, and Plant-Based Protein Powder.

- Probiotic: Vegan coconut or almond yogurt.

Lunch:

- Avocado and Black Bean Salad with Lime Vinaigrette.

- Prebiotic: Sliced radishes.

- Probiotic: Vegan miso soup.

Dinner:

- Stuffed Acorn Squash with Quinoa, Chickpeas, and Roasted Brussels Sprouts.

- Prebiotic: Sliced onions.

- Probiotic: Vegan sauerkraut.

Snack:

- Mixed Berries with a Handful of Almonds.

DAY 40: BREAKFAST:

- Smoothie with Spinach, Mixed Berries, and Plant-Based Protein Powder.
- Probiotic: Vegan probiotic supplement.

Lunch:

- Chickpea Salad Lettuce Wraps with Tahini Dressing.
- Prebiotic: Shredded carrots.
- Probiotic: Vegan miso soup.

Dinner:

- Cauliflower Fried Rice with Tofu and Mixed Vegetables.
- Prebiotic: Chopped green onions.
- Probiotic: Vegan coconut yogurt.

Snack:

- Raw Bell Pepper Strips with Hummus.

DAY 41: BREAKFAST:

- Vegan Omelete with Spinach, Tomatoes, and Vegan Cheese.
- Probiotic: Vegan coconut or almond yogurt.

Lunch:

- Zucchini Noodles with Pesto (nutritional yeast, pine nuts, basil).
- Prebiotic: Sautéed garlic.
- Probiotic: Fermented pickles.

Dinner:

- Baked Portobello Mushrooms with Quinoa and Roasted Brussels Sprouts.
- Prebiotic: Sliced onions.
- Probiotic: Vegan sauerkraut.

Snack:

- Apple Slices with Almond Butter.

Feel free to continue adapting and customizing this meal plan based on your preferences and nutritional needs. As always, listen to your body, stay hydrated, and consult with a healthcare professional or a registered dietitian if you have specific health concerns or dietary requirements.

DAY 42: BREAKFAST:

- Almond Flour Waffles with Mixed Berries and a Drizzle of Maple Syrup.

- Probiotic: Vegan probiotic supplement.

Lunch:

- Broccoli and Almond Salad with Lemon-Tahini Dressing.

- Prebiotic: Raw radishes.

- Probiotic: Fermented pickles.

Dinner:

- Stuffed Bell Peppers with Cauliflower Rice, Black Beans, and Salsa.

- Prebiotic: Sautéed onions and garlic.

- Probiotic: Vegan coconut yogurt.

Snack:

- Mixed Berries with a Handful of Walnuts.

DAY 43: BREAKFAST:

- Smoothie with Spinach, Frozen Berries, and Plant-Based Protein Powder.

- Probiotic: Vegan coconut or almond yogurt.

Lunch:

- Lentil and Vegetable Stir-Fry with Cauliflower Rice.

- Prebiotic: Chopped green onions.

- Probiotic: Vegan coconut yogurt.

Dinner:

- Cauliflower Rice Bowl with Tofu and Mixed Vegetables.

- Prebiotic: Sautéed garlic.

- Probiotic: Vegan kimchi.

Snack:

- Celery Sticks with Peanut Butter.

DAY 44: BREAKFAST:

- Chia Seed Pudding made with Almond Milk, topped with Sliced Strawberries and a sprinkle of Flaxseeds.

- Probiotic: Vegan coconut or almond yogurt.

Lunch:

- Stuffed Acorn Squash with Quinoa, Chickpeas, and Roasted Brussels Sprouts.

- Prebiotic: Sliced onions.

- Probiotic: Vegan sauerkraut.

Dinner:

- Zucchini Noodles with Pesto (nutritional yeast, pine nuts, basil).

- Prebiotic: Sautéed garlic.

- Probiotic: Vegan coconut yogurt.

Snack:

- Raw Carrot Sticks with Hummus.

DAY 45: BREAKFAST:

- Vegan Protein Smoothie with Kale, Pineapple, and Plant-Based Protein Powder.

- Probiotic: Vegan probiotic supplement.

Lunch:

- Grilled Portobello Mushrooms with a Quinoa and Vegetable Stuffing.

- Prebiotic: Sautéed garlic.

- Probiotic: Vegan kimchi.

Dinner:

- Lentil and Vegetable Curry with Cauliflower Rice.

- Prebiotic: Chopped green onions.

- Probiotic: Vegan coconut yogurt.

Snack:

- Mixed Berries with a Handful of Almonds.

DAY 46: BREAKFAST:

- Quinoa Breakfast Bowl with Mixed Berries and Almond Butter.
- Probiotic: Vegan coconut or almond yogurt.

Lunch:

- Stuffed Bell Peppers with Quinoa, Black Beans, and Salsa.
- Prebiotic: Chopped green onions.
- Probiotic: Vegan sauerkraut.

Dinner:

- Cauliflower Rice Bowl with Tofu and Mixed Vegetables.
- Prebiotic: Sautéed garlic.
- Probiotic: Vegan coconut yogurt.

Snack:

- Celery Sticks with Peanut Butter.

Feel free to keep adapting the meal plan based on your preferences, and remember to incorporate a variety of nutrient-dense foods to ensure you're getting a well-rounded intake of essential nutrients. If you have specific dietary concerns or health conditions, consulting with a healthcare professional or a registered dietitian is always a good idea for personalized advice.

DAY 47: BREAKFAST:

- Vegan Omelete with Spinach, Tomatoes, and Vegan Cheese.

- Probiotic: Vegan coconut or almond yogurt.

Lunch:

- Zucchini Noodles with Pesto (nutritional yeast, pine nuts, basil).

- Prebiotic: Sautéed garlic.

- Probiotic: Fermented pickles.

Dinner:

- Baked Portobello Mushrooms with Quinoa and Roasted Brussels Sprouts.

- Prebiotic: Sliced onions.

- Probiotic: Vegan sauerkraut.

Snack:

- Apple Slices with Almond Butter.

DAY 48: BREAKFAST:

- Almond Flour Waffles with Mixed Berries and a Drizzle of Maple Syrup.
- Probiotic: Vegan probiotic supplement.

Lunch:

- Broccoli and Almond Salad with Lemon-Tahini Dressing.
- Prebiotic: Raw radishes.
- Probiotic: Fermented pickles.

Dinner:

- Stuffed Bell Peppers with Cauliflower Rice, Black Beans, and Salsa.
- Prebiotic: Sautéed onions and garlic.
- Probiotic: Vegan coconut yogurt.

Snack:

- Mixed Berries with a Handful of Walnuts.

DAY 49: BREAKFAST:

- Smoothie with Spinach, Frozen Berries, and Plant-Based Protein Powder.
- Probiotic: Vegan coconut or almond yogurt.

Lunch:

- Lentil and Vegetable Stir-Fry with Cauliflower Rice.
- Prebiotic: Chopped green onions.
- Probiotic: Vegan coconut yogurt.

Dinner:

- Cauliflower Rice Bowl with Tofu and Mixed Vegetables.
- Prebiotic: Sautéed garlic.
- Probiotic: Vegan kimchi.

Snack:

- Celery Sticks with Peanut Butter.

DAY 50: BREAKFAST:

- Chia Seed Pudding made with Almond Milk, topped with Sliced Strawberries and a sprinkle of Flaxseeds.

- Probiotic: Vegan coconut or almond yogurt.

Lunch:

- Stuffed Acorn Squash with Quinoa, Chickpeas, and Roasted Brussels Sprouts.

- Prebiotic: Sliced onions.

- Probiotic: Vegan sauerkraut.

Dinner:

- Zucchini Noodles with Pesto (nutritional yeast, pine nuts, basil).

- Prebiotic: Sautéed garlic.

- Probiotic: Vegan coconut yogurt.

Snack:

- Raw Carrot Sticks with Hummus.

DAY 51: BREAKFAST:

- Vegan Protein Smoothie with Kale, Pineapple, and Plant-Based Protein Powder.

- Probiotic: Vegan probiotic supplement.

Lunch:

- Grilled Portobello Mushrooms with a Quinoa and Vegetable Stuffing.

- Prebiotic: Sautéed garlic.

- Probiotic: Vegan kimchi.

Dinner:

- Lentil and Vegetable Curry with Cauliflower Rice.

- Prebiotic: Chopped green onions.

- Probiotic: Vegan coconut yogurt.

Snack:

- Mixed Berries with a Handful of Almonds.

Feel free to keep customizing the meal plan based on your preferences and nutritional needs. Incorporating a variety of colorful vegetables, legumes, nuts, and seeds will help ensure a well-rounded and nutrient-dense diet. If you have specific dietary concerns or health conditions, consulting with a healthcare professional or a registered dietitian is always recommended for personalized advice.

DAY 52: BREAKFAST:

- Quinoa Breakfast Bowl with Mixed Berries and Almond Butter.
- Probiotic: Vegan coconut or almond yogurt.

Lunch:

- Stuffed Bell Peppers with Quinoa, Black Beans, and Salsa.
- Prebiotic: Chopped green onions.
- Probiotic: Vegan sauerkraut.

Dinner:

- Cauliflower Rice Bowl with Tofu and Mixed Vegetables.
- Prebiotic: Sautéed garlic.
- Probiotic: Vegan coconut yogurt.

Snack:

- Celery Sticks with Peanut Butter.

DAY 53: BREAKFAST:

- Chia Seed Pudding made with Almond Milk, topped with Sliced Kiwi and Pomegranate Seeds.
- Probiotic: Vegan coconut or almond yogurt.

Lunch:

- Grilled Portobello Mushrooms with a Quinoa and Vegetable Stuffing.
- Prebiotic: Sautéed garlic.
- Probiotic: Vegan kimchi.

Dinner:

- Lentil and Vegetable Curry with Cauliflower Rice.
- Prebiotic: Chopped green onions.
- Probiotic: Vegan coconut yogurt.

Snack:

- Raw Carrot Sticks with Hummus.

DAY 54: BREAKFAST:

- Vegan Protein Smoothie with Kale, Pineapple, and Plant-Based Protein Powder.

- Probiotic: Vegan coconut or almond yogurt.

Lunch:

- Avocado and Black Bean Salad with Lime Vinaigrette.
- Prebiotic: Sliced radishes.
- Probiotic: Vegan miso soup.

Dinner:

- Stuffed Acorn Squash with Quinoa, Chickpeas, and Roasted Brussels Sprouts.
- Prebiotic: Sliced onions.
- Probiotic: Vegan sauerkraut.

Snack:

- Mixed Berries with a Handful of Almonds.

DAY 55: BREAKFAST:

- Smoothie with Spinach, Frozen Berries, and Plant-Based Protein Powder.

- Probiotic: Vegan coconut or almond yogurt.

Lunch:

- Lentil and Vegetable Stir-Fry with Cauliflower Rice.

- Prebiotic: Chopped green onions.

- Probiotic: Vegan coconut yogurt.

Dinner:

- Cauliflower Rice Bowl with Tofu and Mixed Vegetables.

- Prebiotic: Sautéed garlic.

- Probiotic: Vegan kimchi.

Snack:

- Celery Sticks with Peanut Butter.

DAY 56: BREAKFAST:

- Chia Seed Pudding made with Almond Milk, topped with Sliced Strawberries and a sprinkle of Flaxseeds.
- Probiotic: Vegan coconut or almond yogurt.

Lunch:

- Stuffed Bell Peppers with Cauliflower Rice, Black Beans, and Salsa.
- Prebiotic: Sautéed onions and garlic.
- Probiotic: Vegan coconut yogurt.

Dinner:

- Zucchini Noodles with Pesto (nutritional yeast, pine nuts, basil).
- Prebiotic: Sautéed garlic.
- Probiotic: Vegan coconut yogurt.

Snack:

- Apple Slices with Almond Butter.

DAY 57: BREAKFAST:

- Vegan Omelete with Spinach, Tomatoes, and Vegan Cheese.

- Probiotic: Vegan coconut or almond yogurt.

Lunch:

- Zucchini Noodles with Pesto (nutritional yeast, pine nuts, basil).

- Prebiotic: Sautéed garlic.

- Probiotic: Fermented pickles.

Dinner:

- Baked Portobello Mushrooms with Quinoa and Roasted Brussels Sprouts.

- Prebiotic: Sliced onions.

- Probiotic: Vegan sauerkraut.

Snack:

- Apple Slices with Almond Butter.

DAY 58: BREAKFAST:

- Almond Flour Waffles with Mixed Berries and a Drizzle of Maple Syrup.
- Probiotic: Vegan probiotic supplement.

Lunch:

- Broccoli and Almond Salad with Lemon-Tahini Dressing.
- Prebiotic: Raw radishes.
- Probiotic: Fermented pickles.

Dinner:

- Stuffed Bell Peppers with Cauliflower Rice, Black Beans, and Salsa.
- Prebiotic: Sautéed onions and garlic.
- Probiotic: Vegan coconut yogurt.

Snack:

- Mixed Berries with a Handful of Walnuts.

DAY 59: BREAKFAST:

- Smoothie with Spinach, Frozen Berries, and Plant-Based Protein Powder.

- Probiotic: Vegan coconut or almond yogurt.

Lunch:

- Lentil and Vegetable Stir-Fry with Cauliflower Rice.

- Prebiotic: Chopped green onions.

- Probiotic: Vegan coconut yogurt.

Dinner:

- Cauliflower Rice Bowl with Tofu and Mixed Vegetables.

- Prebiotic: Sautéed garlic.

- Probiotic: Vegan kimchi.

Snack:

- Celery Sticks with Peanut Butter.

DAY 60: BREAKFAST:

- Chia Seed Pudding made with Almond Milk, topped with Sliced Strawberries and a sprinkle of Flaxseeds.

- Probiotic: Vegan coconut or almond yogurt.

Lunch:

- Stuffed Acorn Squash with Quinoa, Chickpeas, and Roasted Brussels Sprouts.

- Prebiotic: Sliced onions.

- Probiotic: Vegan sauerkraut.

Dinner:

- Zucchini Noodles with Pesto (nutritional yeast, pine nuts, basil).

- Prebiotic: Sautéed garlic.

- Probiotic: Vegan coconut yogurt.

Snack:

- Raw Carrot Sticks with Hummus.

DAY 61: BREAKFAST:

- Vegan Protein Smoothie with Kale, Pineapple, and Plant-Based Protein Powder.

- Probiotic: Vegan probiotic supplement.

Lunch:

- Avocado and Black Bean Salad with Lime Vinaigrette.

- Prebiotic: Sliced radishes.

- Probiotic: Vegan miso soup.

Dinner:

- Stuffed Bell Peppers with Quinoa, Black Beans, and Salsa.

- Prebiotic: Chopped green onions.

- Probiotic: Vegan sauerkraut.

Snack:

- Mixed Berries with a Handful of Almonds.

Feel free to continue customizing this meal plan based on your preferences and nutritional needs. Incorporating a variety of colorful vegetables, legumes, nuts, and seeds will help ensure a well-rounded and nutrient-dense diet. If you have specific dietary concerns or health conditions, consulting with a healthcare professional or a registered dietitian is always

DAY 62: BREAKFAST:

- Quinoa Breakfast Bowl with Mixed Berries and Almond Butter.
- Probiotic: Vegan coconut or almond yogurt.

Lunch:

- Stuffed Bell Peppers with Quinoa, Black Beans, and Salsa.
- Prebiotic: Chopped green onions.
- Probiotic: Vegan sauerkraut.

Dinner:

- Cauliflower Rice Bowl with Tofu and Mixed Vegetables.
- Prebiotic: Sautéed garlic.
- Probiotic: Vegan coconut yogurt.

Snack:

- Celery Sticks with Peanut Butter.

DAY 63: BREAKFAST:

- Chia Seed Pudding made with Almond Milk, topped with Sliced Kiwi and Pomegranate Seeds.
- Probiotic: Vegan coconut or almond yogurt.

Lunch:

- Grilled Portobello Mushrooms with a Quinoa and Vegetable Stuffing.
- Prebiotic: Sautéed garlic.
- Probiotic: Vegan kimchi.

Dinner:

- Lentil and Vegetable Curry with Cauliflower Rice.
- Prebiotic: Chopped green onions.
- Probiotic: Vegan coconut yogurt.

Snack:

- Raw Carrot Sticks with Hummus.

DAY 64: BREAKFAST:

- Vegan Protein Smoothie with Kale, Pineapple, and Plant-Based Protein Powder.
- Probiotic: Vegan coconut or almond yogurt.

Lunch:

- Avocado and Black Bean Salad with Lime Vinaigrette.
- Prebiotic: Sliced radishes.
- Probiotic: Vegan miso soup.

Dinner:

- Stuffed Acorn Squash with Quinoa, Chickpeas, and Roasted Brussels Sprouts.
- Prebiotic: Sliced onions.
- Probiotic: Vegan sauerkraut.

Snack:

- Mixed Berries with a Handful of Almonds.

DAY 65: BREAKFAST:

- Smoothie with Spinach, Frozen Berries, and Plant-Based Protein Powder.

- Probiotic: Vegan coconut or almond yogurt.

Lunch:

- Lentil and Vegetable Stir-Fry with Cauliflower Rice.

- Prebiotic: Chopped green onions.

- Probiotic: Vegan coconut yogurt.

Dinner:

- Cauliflower Rice Bowl with Tofu and Mixed Vegetables.

- Prebiotic: Sautéed garlic.

- Probiotic: Vegan kimchi.

Snack:

- Celery Sticks with Peanut Butter.

DAY 66: BREAKFAST:

- Chia Seed Pudding made with Almond Milk, topped with Sliced Strawberries and a sprinkle of Flaxseeds.

- Probiotic: Vegan coconut or almond yogurt.

Lunch:

- Stuffed Bell Peppers with Cauliflower Rice, Black Beans, and Salsa.

- Prebiotic: Sautéed onions and garlic.

- Probiotic: Vegan coconut yogurt.

Dinner:

- Zucchini Noodles with Pesto (nutritional yeast, pine nuts, basil).

- Prebiotic: Sautéed garlic.

- Probiotic: Vegan coconut yogurt.

Snack:

- Apple Slices with Almond Butter.

DAY 67: BREAKFAST:

- Vegan Omelete with Spinach, Tomatoes, and Vegan Cheese.

- Probiotic: Vegan coconut or almond yogurt.

Lunch:

- Zucchini Noodles with Pesto (nutritional yeast, pine nuts, basil).

- Prebiotic: Sautéed garlic.

- Probiotic: Fermented pickles.

Dinner:

- Baked Portobello Mushrooms with Quinoa and Roasted Brussels Sprouts.

- Prebiotic: Sliced onions.

- Probiotic: Vegan sauerkraut.

Snack:

- Apple Slices with Almond Butter.

DAY 68: BREAKFAST:

- Almond Flour Waffles with Mixed Berries and a Drizzle of Maple Syrup.
- Probiotic: Vegan probiotic supplement.

Lunch:

- Broccoli and Almond Salad with Lemon-Tahini Dressing.
- Prebiotic: Raw radishes.
- Probiotic: Fermented pickles.

Dinner:

- Stuffed Bell Peppers with Cauliflower Rice, Black Beans, and Salsa.
- Prebiotic: Sautéed onions and garlic.
- Probiotic: Vegan coconut yogurt.

Snack:

- Mixed Berries with a Handful of Walnuts.

DAY 69: BREAKFAST:

- Smoothie with Spinach, Frozen Berries, and Plant-Based Protein Powder.

- Probiotic: Vegan coconut or almond yogurt.

Lunch:

- Lentil and Vegetable Stir-Fry with Cauliflower Rice.

- Prebiotic: Chopped green onions.

- Probiotic: Vegan coconut yogurt.

Dinner:

- Cauliflower Rice Bowl with Tofu and Mixed Vegetables.

- Prebiotic: Sautéed garlic.

- Probiotic: Vegan kimchi.

Snack:

- Celery Sticks with Peanut Butter.

DAY 70: BREAKFAST:

- Chia Seed Pudding made with Almond Milk, topped with Sliced Strawberries and a sprinkle of Flaxseeds.

- Probiotic: Vegan coconut or almond yogurt.

Lunch:

- Stuffed Acorn Squash with Quinoa, Chickpeas, and Roasted Brussels Sprouts.

- Prebiotic: Sliced onions.

- Probiotic: Vegan sauerkraut.

Dinner:

- Zucchini Noodles with Pesto (nutritional yeast, pine nuts, basil).

- Prebiotic: Sautéed garlic.

- Probiotic: Vegan coconut yogurt.

Snack:

- Raw Carrot Sticks with Hummus.

DAY 71: BREAKFAST:

- Vegan Protein Smoothie with Kale, Pineapple, and Plant-Based Protein Powder.

- Probiotic: Vegan probiotic supplement.

Lunch:

- Avocado and Black Bean Salad with Lime Vinaigrette.

- Prebiotic: Sliced radishes.

- Probiotic: Vegan miso soup.

Dinner:

- Stuffed Bell Peppers with Quinoa, Black Beans, and Salsa.

- Prebiotic: Chopped green onions.

- Probiotic: Vegan sauerkraut.

Snack:

- Mixed Berries with a Handful of Almonds.

DAY 72: BREAKFAST:

- Quinoa Breakfast Bowl with Mixed Berries and Almond Butter.

- Probiotic: Vegan coconut or almond yogurt.

Lunch:

- Stuffed Bell Peppers with Quinoa, Black Beans, and Salsa.

- Prebiotic: Chopped green onions.

- Probiotic: Vegan sauerkraut.

Dinner:

- Cauliflower Rice Bowl with Tofu and Mixed Vegetables.

- Prebiotic: Sautéed garlic.

- Probiotic: Vegan coconut yogurt.

Snack:

- Celery Sticks with Peanut Butter.

DAY 73: BREAKFAST:

- Chia Seed Pudding made with Almond Milk, topped with Sliced Kiwi and Pomegranate Seeds.

- Probiotic: Vegan coconut or almond yogurt.

Lunch:

- Grilled Portobello Mushrooms with a Quinoa and Vegetable Stuffing.

- Prebiotic: Sautéed garlic.

- Probiotic: Vegan kimchi.

Dinner:

- Lentil and Vegetable Curry with Cauliflower Rice.

- Prebiotic: Chopped green onions.

- Probiotic: Vegan coconut yogurt.

Snack:

- Raw Carrot Sticks with Hummus.

DAY 74: BREAKFAST:

- Vegan Protein Smoothie with Kale, Pineapple, and Plant-Based Protein Powder.

- Probiotic: Vegan coconut or almond yogurt.

Lunch:

- Avocado and Black Bean Salad with Lime Vinaigrette.

- Prebiotic: Sliced radishes.

- Probiotic: Vegan miso soup.

Dinner:

- Stuffed Acorn Squash with Quinoa, Chickpeas, and Roasted Brussels Sprouts.

- Prebiotic: Sliced onions.

- Probiotic: Vegan sauerkraut.

Snack:

- Mixed Berries with a Handful of Almonds.

DAY 75: BREAKFAST:

- Smoothie with Spinach, Frozen Berries, and Plant-Based Protein Powder.
- Probiotic: Vegan coconut or almond yogurt.

Lunch:

- Lentil and Vegetable Stir-Fry with Cauliflower Rice.
- Prebiotic: Chopped green onions.
- Probiotic: Vegan coconut yogurt.

Dinner:

- Cauliflower Rice Bowl with Tofu and Mixed Vegetables.
- Prebiotic: Sautéed garlic.
- Probiotic: Vegan kimchi.

Snack:

- Celery Sticks with Peanut Butter.

DAY 76: BREAKFAST:

- Chia Seed Pudding made with Almond Milk, topped with Sliced Strawberries and a sprinkle of Flaxseeds.
- Probiotic: Vegan coconut or almond yogurt.

Lunch:

- Stuffed Bell Peppers with Cauliflower Rice, Black Beans, and Salsa.
- Prebiotic: Sautéed onions and garlic.
- Probiotic: Vegan coconut yogurt.

Dinner:

- Zucchini Noodles with Pesto (nutritional yeast, pine nuts, basil).
- Prebiotic: Sautéed garlic.
- Probiotic: Vegan coconut yogurt.

Snack:

- Apple Slices with Almond Butter.

DAY 77: BREAKFAST:

- Vegan Omelete with Spinach, Tomatoes, and Vegan Cheese.

- Probiotic: Vegan coconut or almond yogurt.

Lunch:

- Zucchini Noodles with Pesto (nutritional yeast, pine nuts, basil).

- Prebiotic: Sautéed garlic.

- Probiotic: Fermented pickles.

Dinner:

- Baked Portobello Mushrooms with Quinoa and Roasted Brussels Sprouts.

- Prebiotic: Sliced onions.

- Probiotic: Vegan sauerkraut.

Snack:

- Apple Slices with Almond Butter.

Feel free to continue customizing this meal plan based on your preferences and nutritional needs. Incorporating a variety of colorful vegetables, legumes, nuts, and seeds will help ensure a well-rounded and nutrient-dense diet. If you have specific dietary concerns or health conditions, consulting with a healthcare professional or a registered dietitian is always recommended for personalized advice.

Prebiotic foods are rich in fibers that promote the growth and activity of beneficial bacteria (probiotics) in the gut. Here is a list of prebiotic foods:

1. **Vegetables:**
   - Asparagus
   - Garlic
   - Onions
   - Leeks
   - Jerusalem artichokes
   - Chicory root
   - Dandelion greens
   - Jicama
   - Radicchio
   - Green bananas

2. **Fruits:**
   - Bananas (under-ripe)
   - Apples
   - Berries (especially strawberries)
   - Kiwi
   - Watermelon
   - Grapefruit
   - Oranges
   - Nectarines
   - Pomegranate

3. **Whole Grains:**

- Oats
- Barley
- Quinoa
- Whole wheat
- Whole grain rice
- Sorghum

4. **Legumes:**
   - Lentils
   - Chickpeas
   - Black beans
   - Kidney beans
   - Navy beans
   - Green peas

5. **Nuts and Seeds:**
   - Almonds
   - Walnuts
   - Pistachios
   - Flaxseeds
   - Chia seeds

6. **Root Vegetables:**
   - Sweet potatoes
   - Carrots

7. **Tubers:**
   - Yams
   - Potatoes

8. **Other:**

- Cocoa (dark chocolate)
- Honey (raw, unprocessed)

It's essential to include a variety of these prebiotic foods in your diet to support a healthy gut microbiome. Combining prebiotic-rich foods with probiotic-rich foods (such as fermented foods like yogurt, kefir, sauerkraut, and kimchi) can contribute to overall gut health. As with any dietary changes, it's advisable to introduce these foods gradually to allow your digestive system to adapt. If you have specific health concerns or conditions, consulting with a healthcare professional or a registered dietitian is recommended for personalized advice.Probiotic foods contain live beneficial bacteria that can contribute to a healthy gut microbiome.

Here is a list of probiotic-rich foods:

1. **Yogurt:**
   - Look for varieties that contain live and active cultures. Choose plain, unsweetened yogurt to avoid added sugars.

2. **Kefir:**
   - A fermented milk product that is similar

to yogurt but has a thinner consistency. It can be dairy or plant-based.

3. **Sauerkraut:**
   - Fermented cabbage that is rich in probiotics. Choose the unpasteurized variety for maximum benefits.

4. **Kimchi:**
   - A Korean dish made from fermented vegetables, usually cabbage and radishes, seasoned with chili peppers and other spices.

5. **Miso:**
   - A traditional Japanese seasoning produced by fermenting soybeans with salt and koji (a type of fungus). It is often used to make miso soup.

6. **Tempeh:**
   - A fermented soy product that originated in Indonesia. It has a firm texture and a nutty, earthy flavor.

7. **Natto:**
   - Fermented soybeans, often eaten in Japan. It has a strong flavor and sticky texture.

8. **Pickles (in brine):**
   - Pickled cucumbers, beets, or other

vegetables that are fermented in brine (salt and water). Look for varieties that have not been pasteurized.

9. **Traditional Buttermilk:**

   - The liquid left behind after churning butter. It is different from the cultured buttermilk commonly found in supermarkets.

10. **Lassi:**

    - A traditional Indian drink made with yogurt, water, and spices. It can be sweet or savory.

11. **Fermented Cheeses:**

    - Certain types of cheese, such as Gouda, cheddar, and Swiss, can contain live cultures.

12. **Traditional Ethiopian Injera:**

    - A sourdough flatbread that undergoes fermentation, often used as a staple in Ethiopian cuisine.

13. **Sourdough Bread:**

    - Bread made with a natural yeast culture, providing a source of probiotics. Look for varieties with a longer fermentation process.

14. **Acidophilus Milk:**

    - Milk fermented with the bacteria Lactobacillus acidophilus.

15. **Probiotic Supplements:**
- Probiotic supplements are available in various forms, including capsules, tablets, and powders. It is important to choose a high-quality supplement with strains that have been researched for their health benefits.

When incorporating probiotic foods into your diet, it is essential to choose options that fit your dietary preferences and needs. If you have specific health concerns or conditions, consulting with a healthcare professional or a registered dietitian is recommended for personalized advice.

Let us Just Recap on all these delicious foods!

Butyrate is a short-chain fatty acid produced by the fermentation of dietary fibers in the colon. It plays a crucial role in maintaining the health of the gut lining and supporting overall gut health. Here is a list of foods that either contain butyrate or contribute to its production in the intestines:

1. **Dietary Fiber-Rich Foods:**
   - Whole grains (oats, barley, brown rice)
   - Legumes (lentils, chickpeas, black beans)
   - Fruits (apples, bananas, berries)
   - Vegetables (broccoli, Brussels sprouts, carrots)
   - Nuts and seeds (flaxseeds, chia seeds, almonds)

2. **Resistant Starch:**
   - Green bananas

- Cooked and cooled potatoes
- Legumes
- Whole grains

3. **Prebiotic Foods:**
    - Garlic
    - Onions
    - Leeks
    - Asparagus
    - Jerusalem artichokes
    - Chicory root
    - Dandelion greens

4. **Fermented Foods:**
    - Fermented dairy products (yogurt, kefir)
    - Sauerkraut
    - Kimchi
    - Miso
    - Tempeh

5. **Butyrate Supplements:**
    - Sodium butyrate supplements are available, but it's important to consult with a healthcare professional before considering any supplementation.

6. **Animal Products:**
    - Grass-fed butter and ghee: While primarily a source of saturated fats, butter contains small amounts of butyrate.
    - Cheese: Some types of cheese may contain trace amounts of butyrate.

7. **Foods Rich in Butyric Acid:**
   - Certain oils, such as butter and ghee, contain butyric acid, which is a precursor to butyrate in the intestines.

8. **Fiber Supplements:**
   - Psyllium husk
   - Inulin supplements

It is important to note that while consuming foods rich in butyrate precursors can support its production in the intestines, individual responses may vary. Additionally, the gut microbiota composition plays a significant role in the production of butyrate. Maintaining a diverse and balanced gut microbiome through a varied and fiber-rich diet is crucial for optimal butyrate production.

As always, if you have specific dietary concerns or health conditions, it is advisable to consult with a healthcare professional or a registered dietitian for personalized advice.

I hope that you enjoyed reading this valuable information that I have provided to you today.

Thank you so much for your support and happy

Gut Healing Revolution: Harnessing the Power of Prebiotics, Probiotics, and Butyrate for Optimal Health and Vitality!

www.ingramcontent.com/pod-product-compliance
Lightning Source LLC
Chambersburg PA
CBHW070948260726
48661CB00003B/1186